Yoga
For
Menstruation

Monique Joiner Siedlak

OSHUN
PUBLICATIONS

Printed in the United States of America

Second Edition 2018

ISBN-13: 978-1-948834-48-3

Publisher
www.oshunpublications.com

Disclaimer
All the material contained in this book is provided for educational and informational purposes only. No responsibility can be taken for any results or outcomes resulting from the use of this material. While every attempt has been made to provide information that is both accurate and effective, the author does not assume any responsibility for the accuracy or use/misuse of this information.

Yoga Poses Photos

Pixabay.com

Freepik.com

Dreamstime.com

Cover Design by Monique Joiner Siedlak

Cover Image by Pixabay.com

Logo Design by Monique Joiner Siedlak

Logo Image by Pixabay.com

Sign up to email list: www.mojosiedlak.com

Other Books in the Series

Yoga for Beginners

Yoga for Stress

Yoga for Back Pain

Yoga for Weight Loss

Yoga for Flexibility

Yoga for Advanced Beginners

Yoga for Fitness

Yoga for Runners

Yoga for Energy

Yoga for Your Sex Life

Yoga: To Beat Depression and Anxiety

Table of Contents

Introduction

That time of the month rolls around and brings with it those pains that make your life a living hell. Menstrual pains are just a great inconvenience and can ruin a week of your life at a time. Over 80 percent of women worldwide face extreme period pains that render them completely unable to move for days. It is important to realize what causes these pains and more important to know how they can be relieved. Medications will only do you so much but there are many other remedies you can do or take that will help you just as if not more.

The most effective exercise proven to help with pains associated with menstrual pains is Yoga. Yoga positions help with relieving pain by stretching out the muscles where the pains are centered. These types of pain however can only be alleviated if positions are held for an extended period of time.

Butterfly Pose (Baddha Konasana)

The Butterfly Pose is a seated pose that strengthens and opens your hips and groin while decreasing abdominal pain.

How to Do

Sit with your knees near to your chest. Relax your knees out to each side and slightly press the bottoms of your feet together. Hold on to your ankles or feet.

Benefits

The Butterfly Pose is a good stretch for your inner thighs, groins, and knees. It helps improve the flexibility in your groin and hip area. When standing and walking for long hours, it removes fatigue.

Can give assistance from menstrual discomfort and menopause symptoms and smooth delivery if it's practiced on a regular basis until late pregnancy. Also helps in intestine and bowel movement.

Tips

You may find it difficult to lower your knees toward the floor. If your knees are incredibly high and your back is rounded, be sure to sit on a high support, even as high as a foot off the floor.

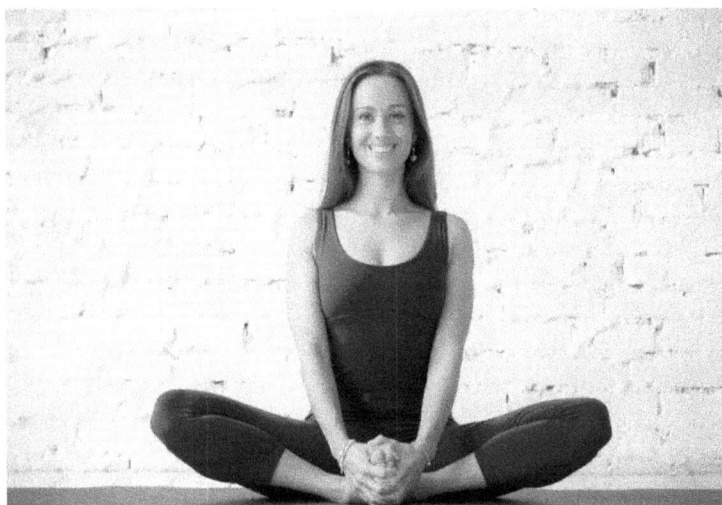

Seated Wide Angle Forward Fold Pose (Upavistha Konasana)

The Seated Wide Angle Forward Fold Pose is a seated yoga pose that deeply elongates your legs and spine, at the same time as calming your mind and releasing stress. It is commonly practiced just before the close of a yoga class, while your body is warm, to get ready your body for even deeper forward bends.

How to Do

Beginning from the Staff Pose, open your legs out as wide as it is comfortable for you. Keep your thighs engaged and your feet arched.

Make sure that your toes are pointing perpendicular to the ceiling as that is the best position for your hips and knees. Don't allow your feet to droop inward or open outward. Press your legs down into the floor.

Breathe in and position down by way of your bottom. Breathe out and forward bend by moving your pelvis forward. Maintain this repetition on each inhale and exhale to deepen the pose.

Let your arms come straight out in front of you and keep your stare softy at the floor to prevent turning your neck.

Benefits

Stimulates your abdominal organs, strengthens the back, stretches your inner thighs and hamstrings and soothes your nervous system.

Tips

Seated Wide Angle Forward Fold Pose is a challenging forward bend for many beginners. If you have trouble bending even a fraction forward, it's okay to bend your knees to some extent. You may possibly even support your knees on rolled blankets or supports; just remember, as you start into the forward bend, it's still essential to keep your kneecaps pointing upwards.

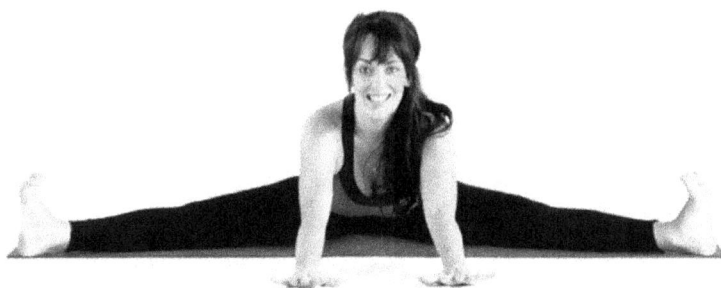

Seated Forward Fold Pose
(Paschimottanasana)

The Seated Forward Fold is a calming yoga pose that aids to relieve stress. This pose is frequently performed later in a series, when the body is warm.

How to Do

From the Staff Pose, inhale the arms up over the head and lift and lengthen up through the fingers and crown of the head. Exhale and bend at the hips, slowly drop your torso towards your legs. Reach the hands to the toes, feet or ankles.

To deepen the stretch, use the arms to gently pull the head and torso closer to the legs. Press out through the heels and gently draw the toes towards you. Breathe and hold for five to ten breaths. To release from this pose slowly roll up the spine back into Staff pose. Inhale the arms back over your head as you lift the torso back into the Staff pose.

Benefits

The Seated Forward Fold delivers a deep stretch for the whole back side of your body from the heels to the neck. The Forward Fold soothes your nervous system and emotions.

Tips

By no means should force yourself into a forward bend, particularly when sitting on the floor. Extend forward, when you feel the area between your pubis and navel shortening, you should stop, lift up a little, and lengthen again. Frequently, because of the tightness in the backs of your legs, a beginner's forward bend doesn't go very far forward and may possibly look more like sitting up straight.

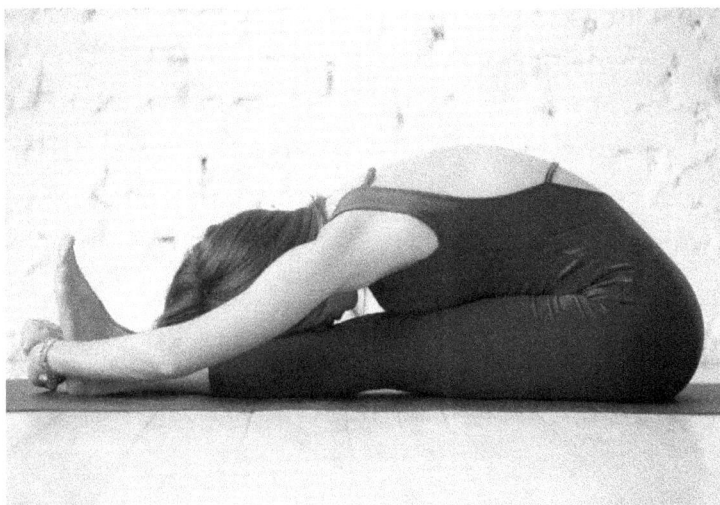

Goddess Pose (Supta Baddha Konasana)

The Goddess Pose, commonly known as the Victory Pose, is a mixture of stretch, physical intensity, and mental power. The Goddess Pose is a wide squat that works the quads and glutes.

How to Do

Starting in the Mountain Pose, separate your feet out roughly three feet wide and parallel, to your mat. Turn your toes out, your heels in, producing a 45-degree angle with both feet.

As you exhale, take a bend deep in your knees, move toward bringing your thighs equal to the floor and your hips aligned with your knees. Your knees will have the inclination to bow in as they bend, so make sure that your knees stay fixed precisely over your ankles.

Spread your arms out at shoulder height and with your palms facing away from you; bend your elbows to 90 degrees. Spread your fingers wide and pull your shoulder blades into your back. Maintain an engaged core and draw your lower ribs into your body. Elongate your tailbone down to the floor and keep your shoulders set precisely over your hips.

Push down evenly across the soles of both feet and continue in the pose for up to five deep breaths.

To release from the pose, extend your legs, lower your arms and step back to Mountain Pose.

Benefits

The Goddess Pose opens your hips and chest at the same time as toning and firming the lower body.

Tips

Bend your knees as much as it seems comfortable to your body. This pose is not suggested for individuals with ankle, knee, or hip conditions.

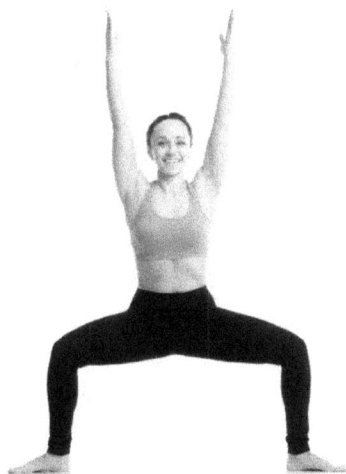

Bow Pose (Dhanurasana)

The Bow Pose is an invigorating pose in which the practitioner lays on their belly, grabs their feet, and lifts the legs into the shape of a bow.

How to Do

Lie on your stomach (prone) with your arms by your side and palms facing upwards. Roll your shoulders on your back so that the tops of your arm bones rise off the floor and your shoulder blades move towards each other. Bend both your knees so that your feet move towards your buttocks.

Clasp your ankles with your hands. You can arch your feet to make a handle. You do not want hold your foot itself. Breathe out and tighten through your abdominal area with the principle of lengthening your lower back and bring support to your spine. Breathe in and lengthen out through the top of your head, while, at the same time, maintaining your knees hip width apart, press your feet back into your hands, forming a natural lift.

With each breath, press your heels back and up, gradually increasing the back bend, keeping the spine elongated. Maintain the effective contraction of the abdominal muscles to counter any pressure that may go into the lower spine.

Hold for 5 breaths or more. Exhale and slowly release the feet. Lie quietly for a few moments. You can repeat if desired.

Benefits

The Bow Pose strengthens your abdominal muscles, adds greater flexibility to the back. It tones the leg and arm muscles, opens up the chest, neck, and shoulders and it is also a useful stress and fatigue buster.

Tips

Place a firm blanket or pillow underneath your hip bones for extra padding, if you need it. To prevent ankle, knee, and other leg injuries, hold onto your ankles, not the tops of your feet.

If it isn't possible for you to clasp your ankles completely, use a strap around the fronts of your ankles and fasten the free ends of the strap, as you maintain your arms fully stretched out.

Remember to keep breathing throughout the pose. Do not hold your breath.

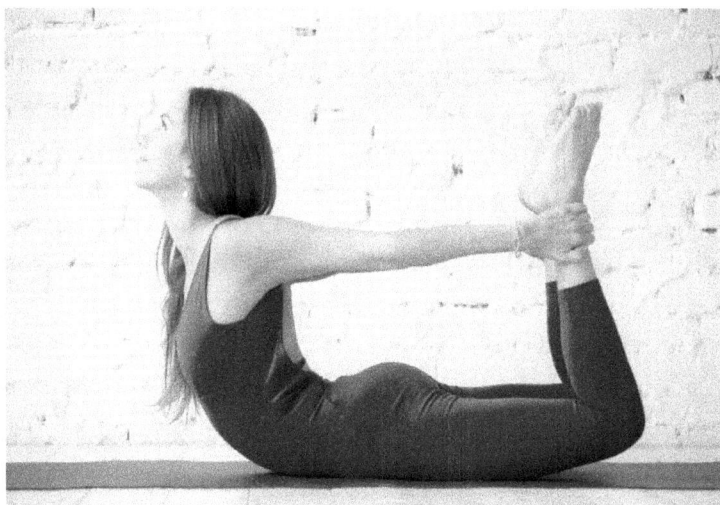

Bridge Pose (Setu Bandha Sarvangasana)

The Bridge Pose is a beginning backbend that helps to open your chest and stretch your thighs.

How to Do

To begin, lie supine (on your back). Fold your knees and keep your feet hip distance apart on the floor, ten to twelve inches from your pelvis, with your knees and ankles in a straight line. With your arms beside your body, place your palms faced down.

Breathe in, while slowly lifting your lower back, middle back and upper back off the floor. Gently roll in your shoulders. Touch your chest to your chin without bringing the chin down. Support your weight with your shoulders, arms, and feet. Feel your buttocks firm up in this pose. Both your thighs should be parallel to each other and to the floor.

You could interlock your fingers and push your hands on the floor to lift your torso a bit more up if you want or you could support your back with your palms. Keep breathing easily.

Hold this pose for a minute or two and then exhale as you gently release the pose.

Benefits

The Bridge Pose strengthens your back, opens the chest, and improves your spinal mobility.

Tips

After you roll your shoulders under, be sure not to pull them away from your ears. This often overstrains your neck. Raise the tops of your shoulders toward your ears and push your inner shoulder blades away from your spine.

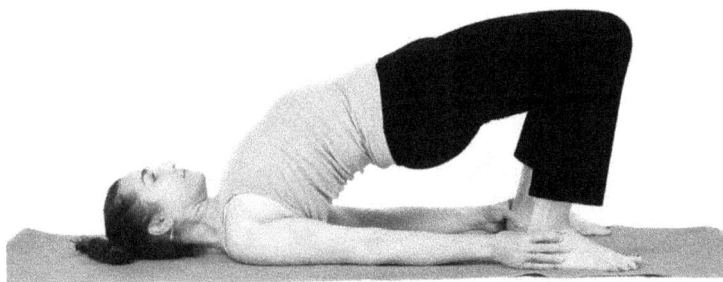

Camel Pose (Ustrasana)

The Camel Pose is an intermediate level back-bending yoga. This yoga posture adds flexibility and strength to the body and also helps in improving digestion.

How to Do

Kneeling on the floor, place your knees hip-width apart and set your hips over the knees. Use a folded blanket if your knees or ankles have aches due to the floor to kneel on. Ground the pose by slightly pushing the top of your feet into the floor.

Lightly tighten your lower abdomen to lean your tailbone down; this will draw your hip points somewhat up towards the bottom of your front ribs. Avoid having stiffness in your buttocks and outer hips while holding this pelvic tilt.

As you maintain a light steadiness in your abdomen, set your hands on the back of your pelvis. The bottom of your palms should go across the tops of your buttocks allowing your fingers to point down. Urge your lower back to lengthen as your tailbone moves deeper into a pelvic tilt as though it is drawing forward toward your pubis. In the course of this action, you should also feel your bottom front ribs slightly being contained as a result adding to the length through your lower back.

Continuing into the back arch, breathe in and roll your shoulders back by pressing your shoulder blades back and against your back ribs. Your chest will inflate and lift. Maintain your pelvis forward over your knees and somewhat lean back against the firmness of the tailbone and shoulder blades.

Remain in this only if you feel relaxed and strong, by slightly twisting to one side to smoothly place one hand on the back of the one heel. Return the spine to center to place the other hand on the other heel. Still keeping the firmness and energy in the abdomen, gently press your thighs forward to perpendicular if the hips have moved back relative to the knees.

Lightly contain the bottom front ribs and continue to lift your hip points towards those ribs to reduce compression of your lower back. Your hands may be positioned so that your palms are on the heels and the fingers point over the soles of the feet. This will allow your upper arm to more effectively externally rotate and add to the expansion of your shoulders and chest. You can continue the pose with the gaze forward. A more advanced version, you can relax the neck and jaw as you gently float your head back. Relax and soften your throat as much as possible-opening the mouth will reduce muscle tension in the front of the neck. Hold the pose with comfort and ease of breath for twenty seconds to a minute.

To release this pose, breathe out and tighten your abdominal muscles. Little by little bring your hands on top of the back of your pelvis one at a time. As you breathe in, tighten your abdominal muscles more to pull your bottom ribs forward causing your trunk to flex forward. Continue to lift your chest over your knees. If your head is back, wait for your chest pass over your knees. At that point let your head flow forward with gravity to avoid strain to the neck. Move slowly into the Child's Pose and rest for a few breaths taking breaths deep into your back.

Benefits

The Camel Pose stretches the front of your body, for the most part, the abdomen, chest, quadriceps, and hip flexors. It improves your spinal flexibility, at the same time as also strengthening your back muscles and improving your posture.

Tips

Beginners very frequently aren't capable to touch their hands to their feet without injuring their back or even their neck. To start with, attempt to turn your toes under and raise your heels. Follow by resting each hand on a block.

Place the blocks just outside each heel, and position them at their highest height. If you're still experiencing difficulty, obtain a chair. Kneel for the pose with your back to the chair, with your calves and feet beneath the seat and the front edge of the seat touching your buttocks. Afterward lean back and bring your hands to the sides of the seat or high up on the front chair legs.

You can also to place a cushion under your knees to assist your way into the pose.

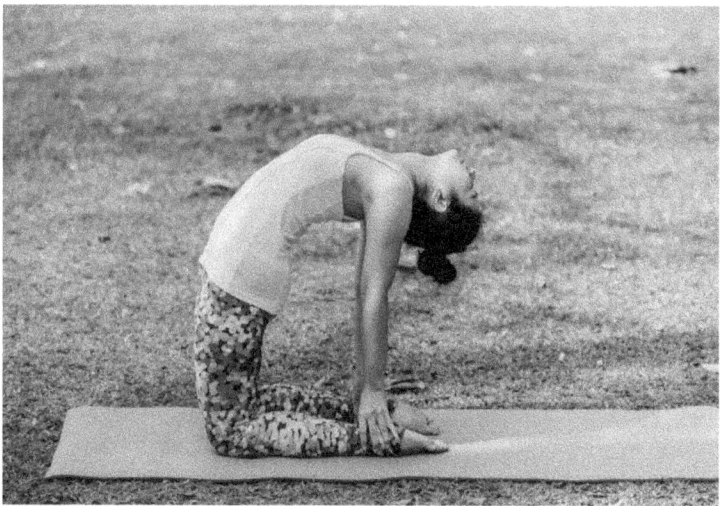

Dolphin Pose (Makarasana)

This intermediate pose will benefit those that are trying to get to headstands.

How to Do

From the Table Pose, lower your forearms to the floor folding the toes under and lift your hips upward to the ceiling. With the middle finger facing forward, spread the fingers wide apart, and your palms shoulder-width apart. Push the forearms, fingers and the palms into the floor, and push your hips up and back. Keeping the spine straight and long, reach up high by way of the tailbone.

Keep your feet at hip's width with the toes facing forward. Push the heels into the floor experiencing a stretch in the back of the legs. You can have a small bend at the knees to keep the back flat or your legs straight. Allow the head and neck fall freely from the shoulders; your forehead can rest on the floor.

Take breaths and hold for two to five breaths. To release this pose, come all the way down to Child's Pose or bend your knees and lower the hips back to the Table Pose.

Benefits

Dolphin is great for improving the upper body, with additional advantages include toning the arms, opening the shoulders, developing hip flexibility and strengthening the abdominals and back muscles.

Open your shoulders by lifting your elbows on a rolled-up sticky mat and pressing your inner wrists firmly to the floor.

Tip

Novices can raise their elbows while doing the Dolphin Pose along with keeping their wrists pushed into the floor. This can help in opening up the shoulders minus any extra stress. To reduce strain on the neck region you can support the head with the use of a pillow or folded blanket.

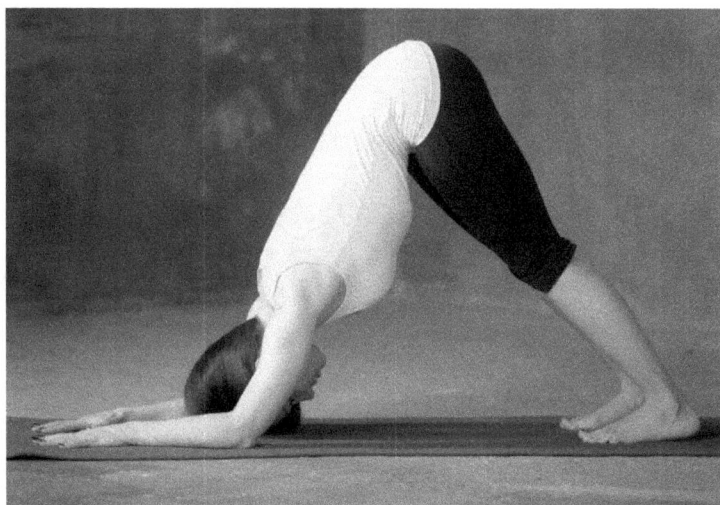

Downward Facing Dog Pose (Adho Mukha Svanasana)

Downward Facing Dog Pose is one of the traditional Sun Salutation sequences poses. It's also an excellent yoga asana all on its own.

How to Do

Begin with your hands and knees in a tabletop position. Make sure your shoulders are aligned above your wrists and your hips are aligned above your knees. Come to a flat back by lengthening the spine. Place your head and neck in a non-aligned position, staring down in the direction of the floor.

Breathe out and raise your knees away from the floor. At the start, keep your knees slightly bent and your heels lifted away from the floor. Lengthen your tailbone positioned from the back of your pelvis and press it slightly toward the pubis. Alongside this tension, raise the resting bones in the direction of the ceiling, and from your inner ankles pull the inner legs up into the groin.

Followed by letting your breath out, push your top thighs back and extend your heels against or down toward the floor. Making sure that you do not lock them, straighten your knees and steady your outer thighs, rolling the upper thighs inward slightly, narrowing the front of the pelvis.

Firming the outer arms, press the bottoms of your index fingers assertively into the floor. From these two points, lift alongside the inside of your arms from the wrists to the tops of the shoulders. Firm your shoulder blades against your back then widen them and draw them toward the tailbone. Keep your head between your upper arms; not allowing it to simply hang.

Continue in this pose somewhere between one to three minutes. Afterward, bend your knees to the floor with a breath and repose in the Child's Pose.

Benefits

Downward Facing Dog pose can help decrease back pain through strengthening the whole back and shoulder girdle. It aids in stronger hands, wrists, the Achilles tendon, low-back, hamstrings, and calves, as well as increasing the full-body circulation. Elongates your shoulders and shoulder blade area. Decrease in tension and headaches by elongating the cervical spine and neck and relaxing the head. It can also lessen anxiety and expand your respiration

Tips

You can alleviate the burden on your wrists by employing a block beneath your palms or you can be capable of completing the pose upon your elbows. By lifting your hands on blocks or the seat of a chair, you can help to release and open your shoulders.

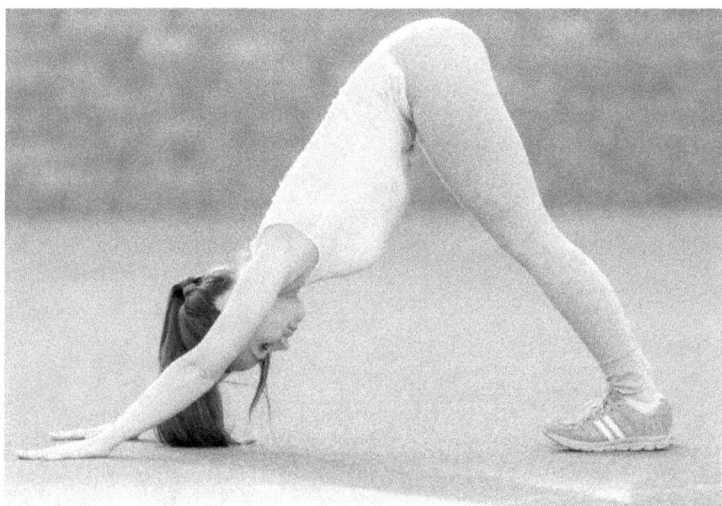

Extended Side Angle Pose (Utthita Parsvakonasana)

The Extended Side Angle Pose is a standing pose that stretches your legs, knees, hips, and ankles while increasing and improving endurance and stamina.

How to Do

Begin in the Mountain Pose. Turn to the right and lengthen your arms sideways to shoulder height with your palms facing down. Move your feet as wide apart as your wrists. Bring into line your heels.

Turn your left leg and foot outward ninety degrees so your toes point to the top of your mat. Bend your left knee until your left thigh is equal to the floor. Keeping your left knee directly over your heel, turn in your right toes to some extent. Line up the heel of your left foot with the arch of your right foot. Keeping your back leg straight, inhale and pull your right hip somewhat forward.

Do not turn your body in the direction of your left leg and keep your torso open to the right. Look out across the top of your left middle finger. This is the Warrior Two pose.

Exhale and lower your left arm so your forearm rests on your left thigh.

Extend your right arm up towards the ceiling, and then spread your arm over the top of your head. Your right bicep must be over your right ear, and your fingertips should be reaching in the same direction with your front toes pointing. Keep your chest, hips, and legs in one straight line, extended over your front leg.

Tilt your head to look up toward the ceiling. Keep your breathing smooth, your throat lax and your face relaxed.

To intensify the pose, lower your front hand to the floor, by placing your palm next to the inside arch of your front foot. Placing your front hand on the outside of your front foot will give you a greater chest and shoulder opening. You can also rest your front hand on a yoga block.

Make certain that your front knee does not drop inwardly. Keeping your front thigh on the outside turning with your knee, drawn it to some extent toward the baby toe of your front foot. Press firmly through the outer edge of your back foot.

Hold for up to one minute.

To release the pose, press firmly across your back foot. Exhale as you slowly rise to a standing position with your arms stretched at shoulder height. Turn your feet and body so they face the same direction, and then move your feet together. Come back to the top of your mat in the Mountain Pose. Repeat on the opposite side.

Benefits

Increases stamina, strengthens while stretching the legs, knees, and ankles.

Tips

Practice with your back heel against a wall or reach your fingers to a yoga block instead of the arch of your foot to make this exercise easier. Don't forget to keep your chest, legs, and hips aligned.

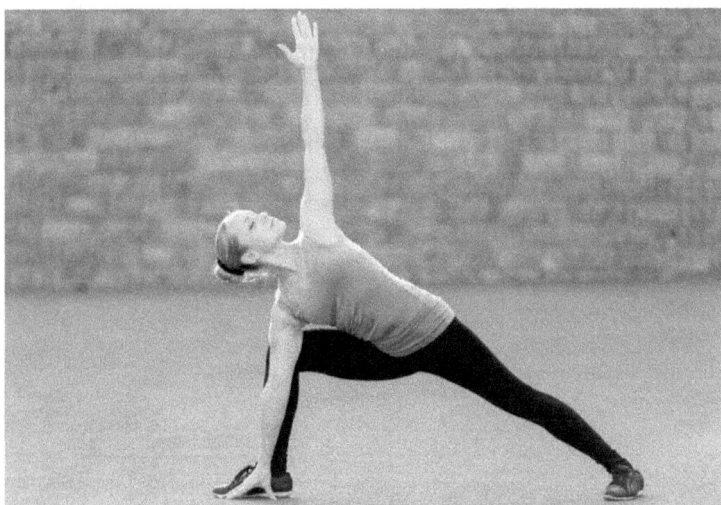

Fish Pose (Matsyasana)

The Fish Pose is performed often as a counterbalance poses to the Shoulder Stand Pose. It stretches your upper body in the opposite way. The Fish Pose has a lot of possibilities because it encourages the throat and crown.

How to Do

Begin by lying on your back. Keeping your feet are together, relax your hands at the side of the body. Inhale. With palms facing down, place the hands underneath your hips. Draw your elbows close to each other and exhale.

Elevate your head and chest, and then inhale. You should extend your legs with your head relaxed back, without adding pressure on your head.

Keeping the chest elevated, lower the head backward and touch the top of your head to the floor. Exhale; allow the chest to open finding awareness of relaxed backbend.

Hold this pose for as long as you can while taking soothing long breaths in and out. With each exhalation, relax in the pose. Raise your head, while lowering your chest and head to the floor. Bring your hands back along the sides of your body and relax.

Benefits

The Fish Pose can help headaches caused by stiffness of the neck. It relaxes Spinal Cord and back muscle tissues. It aids in relieving asthma and respiratory disorders. This yoga pose, when practiced regularly, helps to remedy impotence. Also eases anxiety, mild backache, fatigue and menstrual pain.

Tips

If your head does not comfortably come to the floor, position a blanket or block under your head or slightly lower your chest.

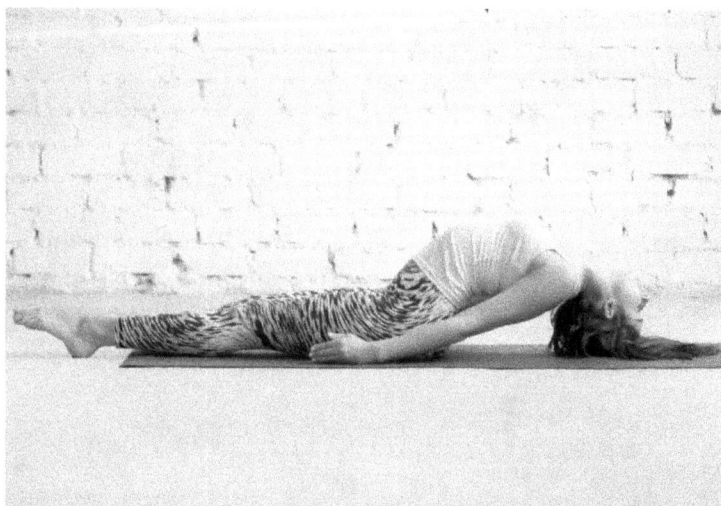

Half Moon Pose (Ardha Chandrasana)

The Half Moon Pose is a standing yoga pose that will test your leg muscles and your capability to balance.

How to Do

Begin by starting in the Extended Triangle Pose to the left side. With your right hand placed on the right hip. breathe in, bending your left knee, and move your right foot about six to twelve inches forward along the floor. Simultaneously, reach your left hand forward, past the little toe side of the left foot, at approximately twelve inches.

While breathing out, push your left hand and left heel firmly into the floor, and straighten your left leg, while at the same time, raising your right leg parallel to the floor. Extend assertively through the right heel to keep the raised leg strong. Make sure the kneecap is aligned straightforward and isn't turned inward and be careful not to lock the standing knee.

Keeping the right hip moving slightly forward, turn your upper torso to the right. Beginners should maintain the right hand on their right hip and their head in a neutral position, staring forward.

Bearing the body's weight mainly on the standing leg, press your lower hand gently to the floor. This will help quickly regulate your balance. As if pulling energy from the floor into the standing groin, lift the innermost ankle of the standing foot strongly upward. Press the sacral region and scapula firmly against the back torso and lengthen the coccyx toward the raised heel.

Remain in this position for thirty seconds to one minute. Drop the raised leg to the floor breathing out, and return to the Extended Triangle Pose. Perform the pose to the right for the same length of time.

Benefits

Increases coordination and equilibrium. Strengthens the abdomen, buttocks, ankles, thighs, and spine. Stretches the shoulders, chest, spine hamstrings and calves,

Tips

Practice with your back foot pressing into a wall or stand in front of a wall to help with balance.

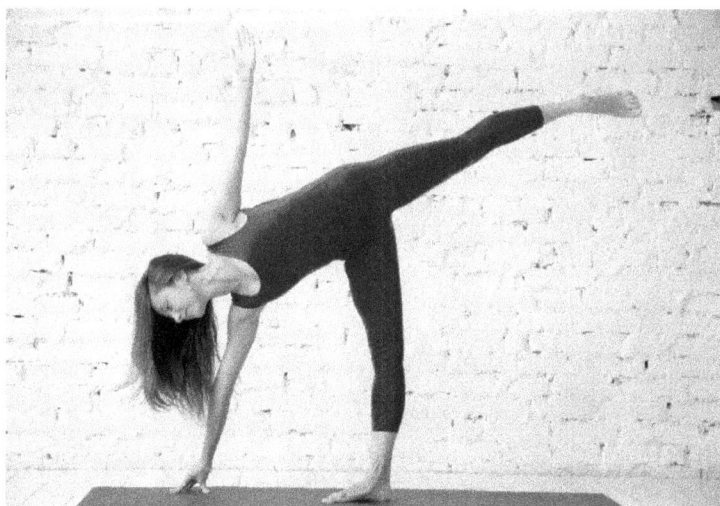

Half Lord of Fishes Pose (Ardha Matsyendrasana)

The Half Lord of Fishes Pose is a moderate to intense twist that encourages length of your spine, a base stretch for your outer hips, and brings forth growth through the chest and shoulders.

How to Do

Begin in a seated position with your legs straight in front of you. Bring in your knees up and bend them with the purpose of your feet are now flat on the floor. This is your beginning position. Bring your right leg beneath your left leg. Maintain your left leg in the starting position. Your right leg should bend at the knee and then keep close to your hip.

Taking your left leg, cross it over the left knee. Set your left foot flat on the floor on the outside of your right knee. Bring your right arm and reach up. Next slowly bend your arm at the elbow and place your elbow on your left knee. Take your left arm and place behind your back and use for a base.

Breathe in and out while either turning your head opposite to the way your back is stretching, or you can turn your head with your back.

Benefits

The Half Lord of Fishes Pose can restore and improve spinal range of motion. It also beneficial for backaches.

Tips

Maintain your right leg extended if you cannot steadily tuck it beneath your left buttock. Squeeze the left knee with your right arm if that feels better than bringing the right elbow outside the left knee. If you normally use a blanket or other prop under your sit bones for seated poses, it's fine to do that here as well.

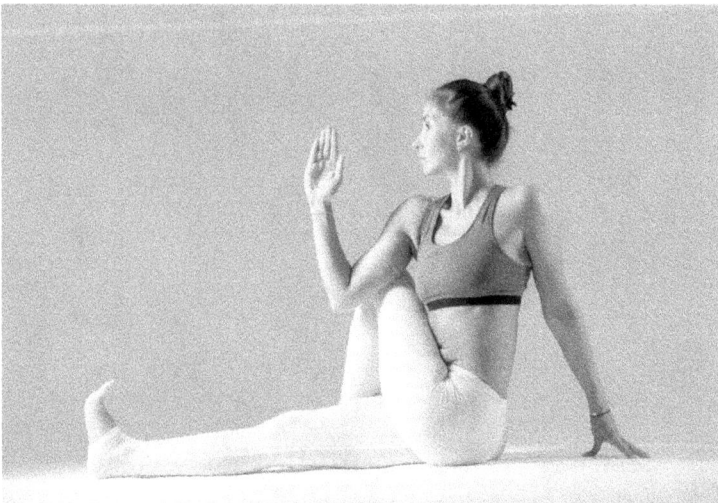

Head-To-Knee Forward Bend Pose (Janu Sirsasana)

The Head-to-Knee Forward Bend Pose is a deep, forward bend that soothes the mind and releases stress. It is frequently practiced near the end of a sequence, when the body is warm, to set up the body for even deeper forward bends.

How to Do

Start in a seated pose with your legs stretched. Bend the right leg, pulling the bottom of the foot to the upper inside of the right thigh. The right knee must rest steadily on the floor. Take both hands to both sides of the left leg. Breathe in and turn towards your extended leg. Breathe out and fold forward. Exhale slowly and deeply for three to five breaths. To come out of the pose, breathe in back to the beginning position. Repeat the other side.

Benefits

Helps tone your legs and burn the fats in your abdominal.

Tip

You can sit up on a blanket if your hips are tight. Place a strap about the extended foot, If you like or hold an end of the strap in each hand as you forward bend.

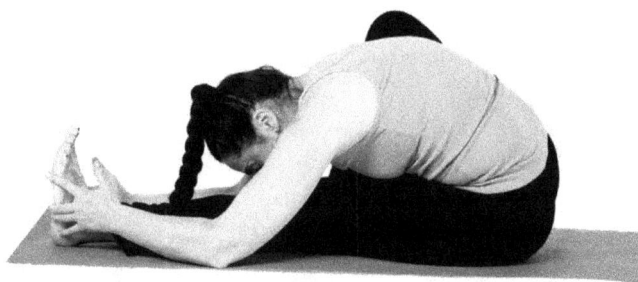

Noose Pose (Pasasana)

The Noose Pose is an advanced binding yoga pose combining a squat and twist where the arms are wrapped around the squatting legs and your hands are clasped behind the back, which forms a noose.

How to Do

Start this pose by standing in the Mountain Pose. You want to bend your knees in such a way you crouch and the buttocks are near to your heels while your upper body is alongside your thighs. You can place a folded blanket, mat or a bolster underneath your heels if you find it tough to squat by setting your feet flat on the floor.

Turn your body from your stomach to the left side. Lengthen your right arm, taking the upper part to the outside of your left knee. Bending your elbow, turn your palm down and wrap your forearm around your left shin.

Lengthen your left arm, in front, curving around and towards the back. Grasp your right wrist in your left hand. You can use a strap to reduce the gap if you find it challenging to perform this. You could also hook your fingers.

Develop the pose by managing the arm that is positioned alongside the knee to twist more, in the direction of the left. To make it easier, turn your head to the left also. Pull your shoulder blades down the back and towards each other.

Make sure that your outer hips are firm and press your heels into the floor, lowering your sitting bones towards them. While breathing in, lift the sternum and lengthen it out, through the top of your head while breathing out, twist your body more, leading with your right ribs

Release the twist after around five breaths. Repeat the exercise with the other side of your body.

Benefits

The Noose Pose stimulates your inner organs. It reliefs aches associated with minor neck, shoulder, back and menstrual pain, and improving posture.

Tip

If you find it difficult for you to get the squatting and the hand movements correct, do it on a chair. Push your right hand against the back of your chair and lift your spine to get a better twist.

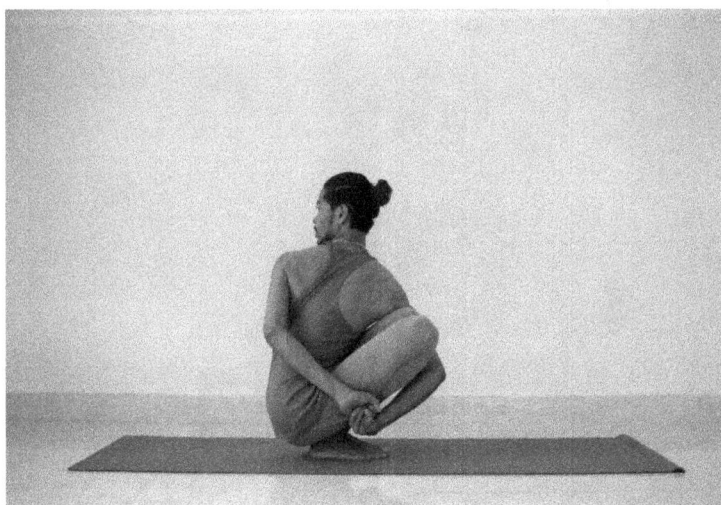

Legs up The Wall Pose (Viparita Karani)

The Legs up the Wall Pose is an upturn pose where you lie on the floor against a wall and position your legs together vertically against the wall.

How to Do

If you are performing the assisted version, place a firm pillow or cushion on the floor against the wall.

Start off the pose by sitting with your right side against the wall. Your lower back should rest against the bolster if you're using one. Slightly turn your body to the right and bring your legs up onto the wall. On the other hand, if you are using a pillow, shift your lower back onto it before bringing your legs up the wall. Use your hands for balance as you transfer your weight.

Drop your back to the floor and lie down. Relax your shoulders and head on the floor. Transfer your weight from side-to-side and move your buttocks close to the wall. Allow your arms to rest open at your sides with your palms facing up. If you're using a pillow, your lower back should at this time be totally held by it.

Allow the part of your bone that connects in the hip socket (the top of your thigh bones) to release and relax, dropping in the direction of the back of your pelvis.

Close your eyes and hold for five to ten minutes, as you breathe with mindfulness.

To release, slowly boost yourself away from the wall and slide your legs down to the left side. Use your hands to help press yourself back up into a seated position.

Benefits

This pose reduces fatigue, cramping in the legs and feet and stretches the back of the legs. It can be an excellent pose for alleviating swollen ankles and calves triggered by long periods of standing pregnancy, and travel. It furthermore elongates the front of the upper body as well as the back of the neck and can be helpful for relieving mild backaches.

Tips

Use your breath to ground the tops of your thighs bones into the wall, which assists in the release of your abdomen, spine, and groins. Imagine in the pose, which each inhalation is falling through your upper body and pushing the tops of your thigh bones closer to the wall. Next with each exhale, hold your thighs to the wall and let your upper body extend over the bolster away from the wall and onto the floor.

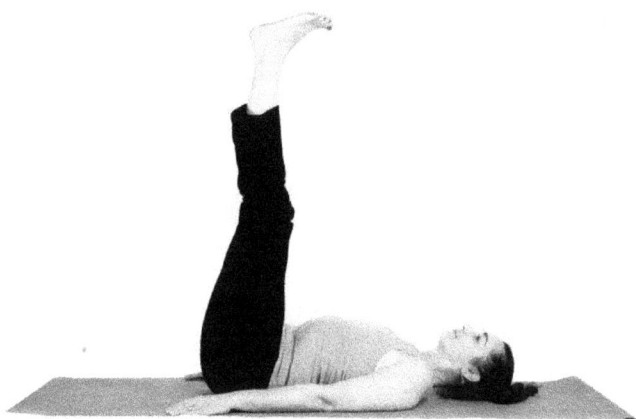

Cobra Pose (Bhujangasana)

The Cobra Pose is a familiar Yoga backbend. When you perform the Cobra Pose, you stretch the front of your torso and spine.

How to Do

Lie face down on the floor. Extend your legs back, with the tops of your feet on the floor. Stretch your hands on the floor beneath your shoulders. Squeeze the elbows back into your body. Push the tops of your feet, thighs, and pubis powerfully into the floor.

On an inhalation, start to straighten your arms to raise your chest off the floor. Go only to a height at which you can sustain a connection throughout your pubis to your legs. Press your tailbone toward the pubis and raise the pubis toward your navel. Narrow the hip, compressing but don't harden your buttocks.

Firm the shoulder blades against the back, puffing the side ribs forward. Lift through the top of the sternum but avoid pushing the front ribs forward, which only hardens the lower back. Distribute the backbend evenly throughout the full spine.

Hold the pose anywhere from fifteen to thirty seconds, breathing freely. Release back to the floor with an exhalation.

Benefits

The Cobra Pose is best known for its capability to build up the flexibility of your spine. It stretches the chest along with strengthening your spine and shoulders. It further assists in opening the lungs and stimulating the abdominal organs, improving digestion.

An energizing backbend, the Cobra Pose can reduce stress and fatigue. It also firms and tones the shoulders, abdomen, and buttocks, and assists in easing back pain.

Tips

The Cobra Pose will be able to energize and warm up the body, getting it ready for the deeper backbends in your yoga routine.

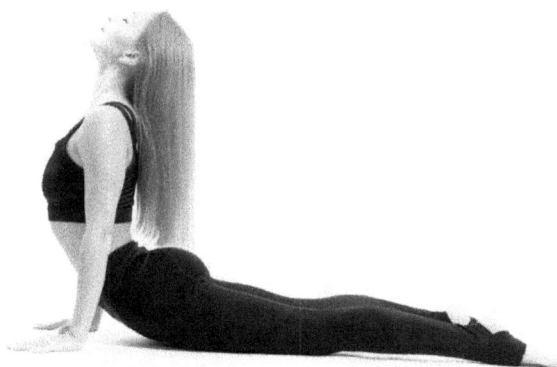

Constructing a Yoga Sequence

Here are a few points to keep in mind how to construct a yoga sequence. You are not at a studio, paying to be there. You do not have to exercise for over an hour. Begin with 5-10 minutes. Notice how you feel by the end of this time. If you feel as if you can do more, go ahead. If no, end your routine there.

Start with 5-10 minutes. By the conclusion of that time, notice how you feel. Do you desire to resume? If yes, continue for an extra five minutes and then check in with yourself once more. If not, close your workout.

The same as any physical journey, a yoga sequence has three clear parts.

Your opening or warm-up sequence

You don't want to jump into the main event tight and cold. This is where you move through and loosening up your major muscle groups as well as body parts

Your main sequence

Once you've warmed up, it's time for your main sequence. This component of your sequence is influenced by the goal of your routine. If it's an asymmetrical pose, keep in mind to do both sides and devote about the same time on each side.

The closing or cool down sequence

Now you've completed the principal portion of your yoga practice, it's time to cool down.

About The Author

Monique Joiner Siedlak is a writer, witch, and warrior on a mission to awaken people to their greatest potential through the power of storytelling infused with mysticism, modern paganism, and new age spirituality. At the young age of 12, she began rigorously studying the fascinating philosophy of Wicca. By the time she was 20, she was self-initiated into the craft, and hasn't looked back ever since. To this day, she has authored over 35 books pertaining to the magick and mysteries of life. Her most recent publication is book one of an Urban Paranormal series entitled "Jaeger Chronicles."

Originally from Long Island, New York, Monique is now a proud inhabitant of Northeast Florida; however, she considers herself to be a citizen of Mother Earth. When she doesn't have a book or pen in hand, she loves exploring new places and learning new things. And being the nature lover that she is, she considers herself to be an avid animal advocate.

To find out more about Monique Joiner Siedlak artistically, spiritually, and personally, feel free to visit her **official website**.

Other Books by Monique Joiner Siedlak

Mojo's Wiccan Series

Wiccan Basics

Candle Magick

Wiccan Spells

Love Spells

Abundance Spells

Hoodoo

Herb Magick

Seven African Powers: The Orishas

Moon Magick

Cooking for the Orishas

Creating Your Own Spells

Body Mind and Soul Series

Creative Visualization

Astral Projection for Beginners

Meditation for Beginners

Reiki for Beginners

Thorne Witch Series

The Phoenix

Beautiful You Series

Creating Your Own Body Butter

Creating Your Own Body Scrub

Creating Your Own Body Spray

Mojo's Self-Improvement Series

Manifesting With the Law of Attraction

Stress Management

Jaeger Chronicles

Glen Cove

Connect With Me!

I really appreciate you reading my book! Please leave a review and let me know your thoughts. Here are the social media locations you can find me at:

Like my Facebook Page: www.facebook.com/mojosiedlak

Follow me on Twitter: www.twitter.com/mojosiedlak

Follow me on Instagram: www.instagram.com/mojosiedlak

Follow me on Bookbub: http://bit.ly/2KEMkqt

Sign up to my Email List at www.mojosiedlak.com and receive a free book!

If you enjoyed this book or found it useful I'd be very grateful if you'd post a short review at your retailer. Your support really does make a difference and I read all the reviews personally so I can get your feedback and make this as well as the next book even better.